Persor

CU00921731

Name: _____

Staff/Stu _____

Health s _____

Health s _____ _

_____

Health service phone number: _____ _____

_____

Useful contact numbers

_____

_____

_____

_____

_____

_____

 Make your own notes with a ballpoint pen and use an alcohol wipe to remove and rewrite.

MIDWIFERY ESSENTIALS

— THIRD EDITION —

MIDWIFERY ESSENTIALS

—— THIRD EDITION —-—

Joanne Gray

Centre for Midwifery, Child and Family Health,
Faculty of Health, University of
Technology Sydney, NSW

Rachel Smith

Centre for Midwifery, Child and Family Health,
Faculty of Health, University of
Technology Sydney, NSW
Burnet Institute
Maternal, Child and Adolescent Health,
Melbourne, Vic

ELSEVIER

ELSEVIER

Elsevier Australia. ACN 001 002 357
(a division of Reed International Books Australia Pty Ltd)
Tower 1, 475 Victoria Avenue, Chatswood, NSW 2067

ISBN: 978-0-7295-4400-9

Notice

Practitioners and researchers must always rely on their own experience
and knowledge in evaluating and using any information, methods,
compounds or experiments described herein. Because of rapid advances
in the medical sciences, in particular, independent verification of
diagnoses and drug dosages should be made. To the fullest extent of the
law, no responsibility is assumed by Elsevier, authors, editors or
contributors for any injury and/or damage to persons or property as a
matter of products liability, negligence or otherwise, or from any use or
operation of any methods, products, instructions, or ideas contained in
the material herein.

National Library of Australia Cataloguing-in-Publication Data

A catalogue record for this
book is available from the
National Library of Australia

NATIONAL
LIBRARY
OF AUSTRALIA

Content Strategist: Libby Houston
Content Project Manager: Fariha Nadeem
Copy Edited by Leanne Peters
Cover by Georgette Hall
Typeset by GW Tech
Printed in Singapore by KHL Printing Co Pte Ltd

Note from the Authors

The authors recognise that individuals have diverse gender identities. Terms such as pregnant person, childbearing people and parent can be used to avoid gendering birth, and those who give birth, as feminine. However, because women are also marginalised and oppressed in most places around the world, we have continued to use the terms woman, mother or maternity. When we use these words, it is not meant to exclude those who give birth and do not identify as women.

CONTENTS

Postnatal period

Newborn baby

General information

Introduction

Midwifery Essentials is a quick reference guide for midwifery students and registered midwives to assist them in their midwifery practice. This guide provides information that is based on current evidence, guidelines and accepted midwifery practice and has a woman-centred approach.

You can personalise this guide to your own particular work setting and then keep this with you to use as a quick reference to inform your practice. Blank pages have been included for you to add information that will assist you in your context of practice.

General principles

This guide is intended as a quick reference and information in the guide is based on the following general principles:

- the provision of woman-centred care
- all care provided should be sensitive to the woman's cultural, social and emotional wellbeing
- all care provided should meet national midwifery practice standards
- every episode of care should involve full discussion with the woman to ensure informed choice, consent and her right to decline
- always consult and follow local policies and protocols.

Schedule of antenatal visits

A schedule of antenatal appointments should be determined according to the function of each appointment. For a nulliparous woman (a woman experiencing her first pregnancy) with an uncomplicated pregnancy, a schedule of 10 appointments should be adequate. For a woman who has had a baby before and has an uncomplicated pregnancy, a schedule of 7 appointments should be adequate. Some women will require more frequent visits, and some women may need fewer visits. It is advisable that women seek pre-conceptual care before planning pregnancy.

The following is a suggested schedule of 10 antenatal visits:

1 Prior to 10 weeks
2 16 weeks (optional)
3 20 weeks
4 26 weeks
5 30 weeks
6 33 weeks
7 36 weeks (from this gestation, some women may benefit from weekly visits)
8 38 weeks
9 40 weeks
10 41 weeks (not always necessary)

(Reference 1.)

Routine antenatal screening

Initial visit (prior to 10 weeks)	**Midwifery assessment**
	· Gestation
	· Social and emotional screening
	· Domestic violence (DV) screening; also referred to as intimate partner violence (IPV), family violence and gender-based violence (GBV)
	· Options of care/planned place of birth discussed
	· Full obstetric, medical, surgical and mental health history
	Routine screening
	· Blood group and antibody screening
	· Body mass index (BMI)
	· Full blood count (FBC)
	· Rubella
	· Hepatitis B
	· Hepatitis C
	· Human immunodeficiency virus (HIV)
	· Syphilis (*Treponema pallidum* haemagglutination/rapid plasma reagin tests)
	· Varicella immunoglobulin G (IgG)
	· Midstream urine test (MSU)
	· Request morphology scan for around 20 weeks
	· Discuss and offer nuchal translucency (NT) ultrasound; NT combined with free beta-human chorionic gonadotrophin and pregnancy-associated plasma protein—A (NTPlus); cell-free DNA testing also known as non-invasive prenatal testing (NIPT) screening, or check results if attended

Continued

(Routine antenatal screening cont.)

	Additional screening as indicated by history **Refer and consult** where appropriate (i.e. genetics, social worker, mental health, obstetric team, etc.)
18–20 weeks	Morphology ultrasound
26–28 weeks	Haemoglobin 75-gm glucose tolerance test (GTT) Antibody screen Discuss and offer anti-D if Rh-negative
34–36 weeks	If indicated: FBC Discuss and offer anti-D if Rh-negative If universal testing: Group B streptococcus (GBS) low vaginal/anal swab

(Reference 1.)

Routine antenatal visit checklist

- Welcome and general enquiry.
- Ask open-ended questions.
- Consider maternal social, emotional and cultural wellbeing.
- Calculate gestation together with woman.
- Assessment of fetal wellbeing:
  - maternal enquiry
  - fetal movements—discuss fetal movement patterns and advise woman to contact midwife/health service if pattern changes/movements decrease
  - fundal height measurement
  - abdominal palpation
  - fetal heart rate auscultation.
- Order and explain any routinely offered tests.
- Discuss and offer any recommended vaccinations.
- Check blood pressure.
- Address concerns or questions.
- Gestation-specific discussions:
  - normal fetal movement patterns
  - common disorders
  - onset of labour
  - pain in labour
  - preparation for birth/breastfeeding.
- Ongoing plan for pregnancy.
- Consultation and referral where indicated.
- Arrange next visit.
- Provide advice/information as required (i.e. breastfeeding, what to expect when labour commences).
- Documentation.

(References 1 and 2.)

Calculating expected date of birth (EDB)

Naegele's rule

- Take woman's menstrual history including average cycle length.
- Note Naegele's rule can only be used when the woman experiences a regular menstrual cycle.

Ultrasound scan (USS) may be used in combination or if dates differ significantly (USS is most accurate in estimating gestation between 8–14 weeks).

Calculation

First day of last normal menstrual period (LNMP)
+ 7 days
+ 9 months
Adjust for cycle length.
Adjustment for cycle length

- If 28-day cycle, no adjustment required.
- If > 28 days, add the number of days over 28 to the final calculated date (i.e. for a 32-day cycle, add 4 days to the EDB).
- If < 28 days, subtract the number of days below 28 from the final calculated date (i.e. for a 25-day cycle, subtract 3 days from the EDB).

Example

Mariam's LNMP was 18 February 2021. She has a 29-day cycle.

LNMP = 18 February 2021
+ 7 days = 25 February 2021
+ 9 months = 25 November 2021
+ 1 day adjustment = 26 November 2021 = EDB

LNMP and USS calculations

If LNMP is certain and menstruation regular, compare estimation to dating USS.

- If USS between 6–13 weeks: if both dates are within 5 days use LNMP date; if more than 5 days' difference use USS date.
- If USS between 13–24 weeks: if both dates differ by 10 days or less use LNMP; if more than 10 days' difference use USS date.

(Reference 1.)

Routine blood tests in pregnancy

Test	Rationale/notes
Full blood count (FBC)	• First trimester baseline • Repeat at 28 weeks • Plasma expansion leads to haemodilution and fall in haemoglobin (Hb) and haematocrit—physiological anaemia • Hb lower than 110 g/L in first trimester or 105 g/L at 28 weeks requires investigation and/or supplementation; consider iron studies
ABO blood group, Rh factor and red cell antibodies	• Identify Rh-negative women who require further antibody testing and should be offered anti-D immunoglobulin at 28 and 34 weeks • Assist in identifying babies at risk of developing haemolytic disease
Rubella antibodies	• Identify immunity to rubella • Prevent congenital rubella syndrome • Offer postpartum vaccine if non-immune or borderline immunity

(Routine blood tests in pregnancy cont.)

Test	Rationale/notes
Syphilis	• VDRL test (venereal disease research laboratory) • RPR/TPHA (rapid plasma reagin/*Treponema pallidium* haemagglutination tests) • Syphilis can result in spontaneous abortion, stillbirth, intrauterine growth restriction and perinatal death
Hepatitis B	• Most commonly transmitted blood-borne virus • Screening identifies immunity, infection and carrier status
Hepatitis C	• Identifies women who have hepatitis C and enables the avoidance of intrapartum invasive procedures that increase risk of transmission • Effective treatments can be offered post birth/breastfeeding
75-g glucose tolerance test (GTT)	• Recommended at 26–28 weeks • If risk factors for diabetes (see Diabetes in Pregnancy) offer glycated haemoglobin (HbA1c) or fasting blood glucose test in the first trimester

Continued

(Routine blood tests in pregnancy cont.)

Test	Rationale/notes
Human immunodeficiency virus (HIV)	• Allow for treatment to reduce perinatal transmission • Recommendation that all pregnant women be offered HIV screening at first visit
Others	Offer other tests depending on population or individual risk factors: • vitamin D • varicella IgG • thyroid function • iron studies • haemoglobin electrophoresis (HbEPG) • bacterial vaginosis • *Chlamydia*

(Reference 1.)

Other screening tests in pregnancy

Test	Rationale/notes
Midstream urine (MSU) for culture and sensitivity	• At first visit • To screen for asymptomatic bacteriuria and offer treatment if present
Low vaginal swab	• Test for Group B streptococcus (GBS) • If positive, follow up as per local policy
Morphology ultrasound	• Recommended that all pregnant women are offered a routine fetal anomaly ultrasound at 18–20 weeks • Identifies anomalies that are incompatible with life; associated with significant morbidity or disability; may benefit from intervention/treatment • Provides options to parents for pregnancy progression

Continued

(Other screening tests in pregnancy cont.)

Test	Rationale/notes
First-trimester screening for chromosomal anomalies	Following discussion with the woman, consider offering: • nuchal translucency (combined) • cell-free DNA/non-invasive perinatal testing (NIPT) • referral to genetic services if indicated
Genetic screening and diagnostic testing	• A number of screening and diagnostic tests are available, including chorionic villus sampling (CVS) and amniocentesis; women may consider having prenatal screening or testing and they should be referred as appropriate

(Reference 1.)

Vital sign measurement—maternal

Many healthcare services now utilise track and trigger systems. These rely on periodic measurement and documentation of vital signs with predetermined actions for when thresholds are reached. There are many different track and trigger systems in use nationally and internationally. This information is based on the modified early obstetric warning system (MEOWS) for New South Wales (Between the Flags). Normal parameters may differ slightly depending on where you work—refer to local policy and initiate local response systems where observations are outside accepted ranges.

Normal blood pressure

Systolic < 140
Diastolic < 90

Temperature

Range 36–37.5°C

Pulse

Range 50–120 beats per minute

Respirations

Range 10–25 breaths per minute

SpO²

Range 95–100%

(Reference 3.)

Korotkoff's sounds

Measurement of blood pressure by auscultation is based on the sounds produced as a result of changes in blood flow, termed Korotkoff's sounds.

Phase I	The pressure level at which the first faint, clear tapping sounds are heard, which increase as the cuff is deflated (reference point for systolic blood pressure)
Phase II	During cuff deflation when a murmur or swishing sounds are heard
Phase III	The period during which sounds are crisper and increase in intensity
Phase IV	When a distinct, abrupt, muffling of sound is heard
Phase V	The pressure level when the last sound is heard (reference point for diastolic blood pressure—use Phase IV if Phase V is absent)

(Reference 4)

Hypertension in pregnancy

Changes to a woman's blood pressure during pregnancy

- Hormonal influences in pregnancy cause decreased vascular resistance. This, coupled with the increase in circulating volume, leads to a marked decrease in the diastolic blood pressure but little change in the systolic blood pressure.
- Blood pressure gradually rises, returning to prepregnant levels by term.

Accurate measurement of blood pressure in pregnancy

- Rested and seated comfortably.
- Feet flat on floor.
- Lateral recumbency (if required).
- If upper arm circumference > 33 cm, use large cuff.
- If upper arm circumference greater than 44 cm, use thigh cuff.
- Use right arm.

Hypertension in pregnancy

Diagnosed when:
- systolic blood pressure is ≥ 140 mmHg *and/or*
- diastolic blood pressure (Korotkoff V) is ≥ 90 mmHg.

Gestational hypertension

This is hypertension arising in pregnancy after 20 weeks without any feature of the multisystem disorder pre-eclampsia, and which resolves within 3 months postpartum.

Pre-eclampsia

This is hypertension arising after 20 weeks' gestation accompanied by one or more of the following:

- **proteinuria**—spot urine protein/creatinine ratio > 30 mg/mmol
- **renal insufficiency**—serum/plasma creatinine > 90 µmol/L or oliguria
- **liver involvement**—raised serum transaminases and/or severe epigastric pain
- **neurological involvement**—convulsions (eclampsia); hyperreflexia with clonus; persistent new headaches; persistent visual disturbances (scotomata); stroke
- **haematological disturbances**—thrombocytopenia < 100 000/µL; haemolysis; disseminated intravascular coagulation
- **pulmonary oedema**—sudden onset of breathlessness, may be accompanied by agitation
- **fetal growth restriction**—indicating placental insufficiency.

Pre-eclampsia blood tests

Tests routinely ordered when diagnosing and/or treating pre-eclampsia (often referred to as PE bloods):

- full blood count (FBC), including platelets
- liver function tests (LFT)
- urea, electrolytes and creatinine (UEC)
- uric acid
- spot urine for protein/creatinine ratio.

(Reference 4.)

Diabetes in pregnancy

This section provides information on diabetes diagnosed during pregnancy (not preexisting type 1 or 2). Diabetes diagnosed in pregnancy can be either previously undiagnosed type 2 diabetes or gestational diabetes (GD).

Assess risk factors for diabetes at the initial visit. Risk factors include:

- advanced maternal age
- increased BMI
- presence of polycystic ovarian syndrome
- previous obstetric history—high birth weight baby; previous unexplained stillbirth; previous GD
- family history of diabetes
- ethnic origin, including: Aboriginal and/or Torres Strait Islander peoples, Māori, Pacific Islands, south and/or east Asian origin.

If risk factors are identified, discuss and offer a glycated haemoglobin (HbA1c) or fasting glucose. Suggested thresholds are as shown below.

| HbA1c | ≥ 4.1 mmol/mol (5.9%) |
| Fasting plasma glucose | 6.1–6.9 mmol/L |

Universal screening for gestational diabetes

Consensus-based recommendations advise offering all women testing for diabetes between 26 and 28 weeks' gestation using the World Health Organization (WHO) and the International Association of Diabetes and Pregnancy Study Groups (IADPSG) diagnostic criteria for gestational diabetes below.

Fasting plasma glucose	5.1–6.9 mmol/L
1-hour plasma glucose	> or = 10.0 mmol/L following a 75-g oral glucose load
2-hour plasma glucose	8.5–11.0 mmol/L following a 75-g oral glucose load

If diabetes is diagnosed, ensure the following:
• full discussion of test results and recommended treatments/management
• referral to appropriate services
• provision of culturally appropriate and respectful information and support to assist women to manage the diabetes
• ongoing follow-up and support.

(Reference 1.)

Abdominal palpation

Aims

* Observe the signs of pregnancy and parity.
* Assess fetal size and growth.
  Detect deviations from normal.
* Determine fetal position and presentation.
  Auscultate fetal heart.

Definitions

Attitude	Relationship of the fetal limbs and head to the fetal trunk (e.g. flexed, extended)
Auscultation	Listening to the fetal heart rate
Denominator	The name of the part of the presentation, used when referring to fetal position (e.g. occiput, sacrum, mentum)
Engagement	Occurs when the widest diameter of the presenting part passes through the brim of the pelvis
Fundal height	Measured in centimetres using a tape measure from the top of the uterus (fundus) to the symphysis pubis
Fundal palpation	Determines the presence of the breech or the head in the uterine fundus

Continued

(Definitions cont.)

Inspection	Assessment by observation
Lateral palpation	Used to locate the fetal back in order to determine position
Lie	The relationship between the long axis of the fetus and the long axis of the uterus (e.g. longitudinal, transverse, oblique)
Palpation	Examination by touch
Pelvic palpation	Identifies the pole of the fetus in the pelvis
Position	The relationship of the denominator of the presentation and six points on the pelvic brim (e.g. left or right—anterior, lateral, posterior)
Presentation	Part of the fetus that lies at the pelvic brim or in the lower pole of the uterus (e.g. cephalic/ vertex, breech, face, brow, shoulder)
Presenting part	Presenting part of the fetus that lies over the cervical os during labour (e.g. cephalic, breech)

(References 5 and 6.)

Diagrams of fetal positions are given over the page in Fig. 1.

Figure 1
Fetal positions—right

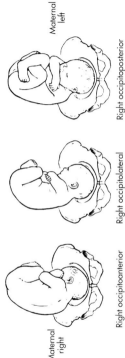

Right occipitoanterior

Right occipitolateral

Right occipitoposterior

Maternal right

Maternal left

(Reference 6.)
Continued

Figure 1
Fetal positions—left

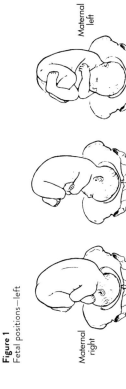

Left occipitoposterior

Left occipitolateral

Left occipitoanterior

Maternal left

Maternal right

(Reference 6.)

Body mass index (BMI)

Calculation and guidelines

$$BMI = \frac{weight\ (kg)}{height^2\ (m^2)}$$

BMI	Category	Recommended weight gain in pregnancy
< 18.5	Underweight	12.7–18.1 kg
18.5–24.9	Desirable	11.3–15.9 kg
25–29.9	Overweight/pre-obesity	6.8–11.3 kg
30–39.9	Obese · Class I: 30–34.9 · Class II: 35–39.9	5–9 kg
> 40	Class III: Obesity	5–9 kg

Note that the BMI can be less accurate for assessing healthy weight in certain groups due to variations in muscle mass and fat mass.

(References 1 and 7.)

Sample calculations

Example 1

Eleni is 173 cm tall and weighs 82 kg.

1.73 × 1.73 = 2.99 (height in metres, squared)

82 ÷ 2.99 = 27.4

Eleni's BMI is 27.4 which puts her in the overweight category.

Example 2

Fenglian is 165 cm tall and weighs 58 kg.

$$1.65 \times 1.65 = 2.72$$

$$58 \div 2.72 = 21.3$$

Fenglian's BMI is 21.3 which puts her in the healthy weight range.

Fetal growth patterns

Gestation	Length (cm)	Weight (grams)	Activities
8 weeks	1.6	1	• Face forming • Arms and legs moving • Fetal heart detectable by ultrasound
12 weeks	5.4	45	• Can suck and swallow • Sex is distinguishable
16 weeks	11.6	240	• Downy hair covers body • Coordinated movements present
20 weeks	16.4	460	• Sucks thumb • Hair, eyelashes and eyebrows are present
24 weeks	30	820	• Eyes are open • Has strong grip
28 weeks	37.6	1300	• Adding body fat • Eyesight developing
32 weeks	42.4	2100	• Periods of sleep and wakefulness • Responds to sounds
36 weeks	47.4	2900	• Skin less wrinkled • May assume birth position
40 weeks	51.2	3400	• Awaiting birth

(Reference 8.)

Consultation and referral

If problems occur during pregnancy or birth, the midwife may consult with peers in the first instance; or consult directly with a secondary- or tertiary-level caregiver and refer when appropriate.

- The consultation and referral level is dependent on the severity of the condition.
- **When there is any doubt, consultation is recommended.**

Any discussion, consultation or referral and subsequent care decisions, recommendations and/or actions should be clearly documented.

Australian College of Midwives (ACM) levels of consultation and referral

Level	Definition	Examples
A or A* **Discuss**	(A): Discussion with another midwife and/ or medical practitioner/ other healthcare provider (A*): Refers to midwives endorsed to prescribe medicines and diagnostic tests	• Breastfeeding difficulties • Suspected deviations from normal • Previous pregnancy problem

(Australian College of Midwives (ACM) levels of consultation and referral cont.)

Level	Definition	Examples
B **Consult**	Consultation and possible transfer or sharing of care	• Use of alcohol or other drugs • Previous history of a baby with congenital or hereditary disorder • Size/date discrepancy • Suspected maternal infection
C **Refer**	Transfer of care (wherever possible the midwife will continue to support the woman)	• Fetal death in utero • Pre-eclampsia • Cardiovascular disease • Postpartum psychosis • Diabetes mellitus • HIV infection

(Reference 2.)

Labour and birth definitions

Augmentation of labour	To accelerate or intensify the process of spontaneous labour
Effacement	The taking-up of the length of the cervical canal into the lower segment of the uterus
First stage of labour	From onset of painful uterine contractions associated with cervical dilation to full dilation of the cervix. Divided into two phases: • **latent**—the early phase of the first stage of labour; in terms of cervical dilation, generally considered from 0–5 cm • **active**—phase when the cervix undergoes more rapid dilation and labour is considered established (from 5 cm—full dilation)
Induction of labour	Intentional stimulation of the pregnant uterus to initiate labour using pharmacological, surgical or mechanical means
Normal labour	Four parameters: • spontaneous in onset • no complications arise • vertex presents • at term—37 completed weeks

Continued

(Labour and birth definitions cont.)

Prelabour	Irregular mild uterine activity associated with some cervical effacement
Preterm	Gestation prior to 37 completed weeks of pregnancy
Second stage of labour	From full dilation of the cervix to the birth of the baby
Term	37 completed weeks of pregnancy and beyond
Third stage of labour	From birth of the baby to expulsion of the placenta and membranes and control of blood loss

(References 6 and 9.)

Mechanism of labour and birth (occipitoanterior position)

Descent	Begins before onset of labour; continues throughout labour and birth
Flexion	Pressure exerted down the fetal axis causes the fetal head to flex so that the chin tucks further onto the fetal chest
Internal rotation of the head	The presenting part meets pelvic floor resistance and rotates; flexion is maintained and the occiput slips beneath the subpubic arch (crowning)
Extension of the head	The head is born by extension; this releases the sinciput and allows face and chin to sweep the perineum
Restitution	The twist in the fetal neck caused by internal rotation of the head now corrects itself; the occiput moves one-eighth of a circle towards the side from which it started
Internal rotation of the shoulders	The shoulders rotate so that they lie in the anteroposterior diameter of the pelvis
Lateral flexion	The shoulders are born sequentially; anterior shoulder usually first with the remainder of the body born by lateral flexion to follow the curve of the pelvis

See Fig. 2 (pp. 34–5) for diagrams.

Figure 2

Descent of the fetal head (A) and dilation of the cervix (B)

A

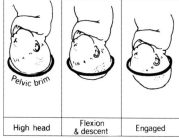

| High head | Flexion & descent | Engaged |

B

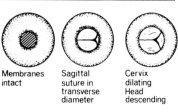

| Membranes intact | Sagittal suture in transverse diameter | Cervix dilating Head descending |

(Figure 2 cont.)

A

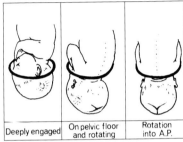

| Deeply engaged | On pelvic floor and rotating | Rotation into A.P. |

B

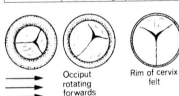

Occiput rotating forwards

Rim of cervix felt

(Reference 6.)

Promoting normal birth

Strategies to promote normal birth should include the following.

1 Provision of continuity of midwifery care

- Builds trusting relationships.
- Reduces intervention in labour and at birth.
- Increases women's feelings of control and satisfaction.

2 Provide a safe birth environment

- Encourage development of a birth plan.
- Ensure and protect privacy.
- Provide low lighting.
- Provide and support use of equipment/props that promote upright and active labour.
- Ensure one-to-one care in labour and at birth.
- Provide a comfortable and individualised environment (own clothes, music, pillows, pictures etc.).

3 Support activity

- Encourage upright and active labour.
- Consider positioning for birth.
- Promote the use of gravity.
- Avoid disturbances to the natural rhythm of labour.

Avoid intervention

Ask if it is really necessary.
No admission cardiotocography (CTG) for low-risk women.
Avoid the 'cascade' of intervention.
Avoid technology unless necessary.
Avoid arbitrary time limits—personalise care.
Ensure a continuous supportive presence.
Avoid early admission to hospital/birth centre in labour—support and encourage women to stay at home.

Ensure continuous practice improvement

- Utilise a process of supported practice review.
- Regularly assess your learning needs and seek development in areas of need.
- Seek out and engage with a midwifery mentor.
- Engage in professional development.
- Join and actively participate in your professional association.

(Reference 10.)

Vaginal examinations

General considerations

- Explain and discuss procedure.
- Gain consent.
- Follow standard precautions.
- Ensure comfort.
- Ensure privacy.

Examination

Perform an abdominal palpation prior to every vaginal examination.

During a vaginal examination you should assess the following.

External genitalia	· Irregularities · Varicosities · Signs of infection
Vagina	· General appearance · Temperature · Lubrication · State of adjacent structures
Cervix	· Position · Consistency · Length · Dilation

Vaginal examinations cont.)

Membranes	• Intact • Presence of forewaters • Colour of liquor
Presentation (see Fig. 3, pp. 40–1)	• Cephalic/breech • Face/brow • Cord • Compound
Station (see Fig. 4, p. 41)	• Level of presenting part in relation to ischial spines (in centimetres above or below the spines)
Position (see Fig. 5, p. 42)	• Position of the suture lines and fontanelles in relation to the maternal pelvis
Pelvic outlet	• Subpubic arch • > 90 degrees?
Fetal heart rate	• Record and document fetal heart rate on completion of vaginal examination

Figure 3
The five presentations

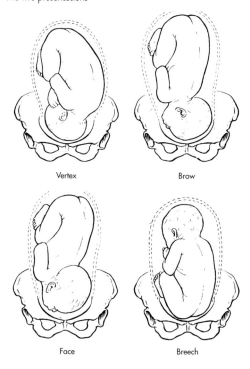

Vertex

Brow

Face

Breech

Figure 3 cont.)

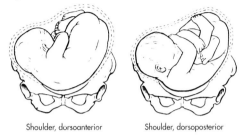

Shoulder, dorsoanterior   Shoulder, dorsoposterior

(Reference 6.)

Figure 4
Stations of the fetal head (measured in centimetres above/
below the spines)

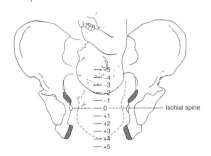

(Reference 11.)

Figure 5
Six positions in vertex presentation,

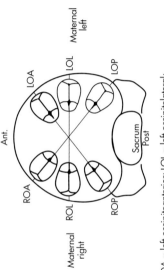

LOA = left occipitoanterior; LOL = left occipitolateral;
LOP = left occipitoposterior; ROA = right occipitoanterior;
ROL = right occipitolateral; ROP = right occipitoposterior.

The cervix in labour

When assessing the cervix in labour, assess and document:

- **position**—anterior, posterior or midway
- **consistency**—firm, moderate, soft, stretchy
- **length** (effacement)—in cm
- **dilation**—in cm
- **application of presenting part**—well applied, poorly applied.

Diagrams of the cervix in labour are given in Fig. 2 (pp. 34 5).

Bishop's score

A vaginal examination is carried out to assess the readiness of the cervix for an induction of labour, using the Bishop's score. The higher the score, the more likely that there can be a successful induction of labour.

Examination findings	Score			
	0	1	2	3
Dilation (cm)	Closed	1–2	3–4	> 5
Length (cm)	3	2	1	0
Station*	−3	−2	1 or 0	+1, +2
Consistency	Firm	Medium	Soft	–
Position of cervix	Posterior	Midposition	Anterior	–

*See Fig. 4 (p. 41) for stations of the fetal head.

(Reference 6.)

Intermittent fetal heart rate auscultation

Women at low risk of complications should be offered intermittent auscultation of the fetal heart rate when in established labour.

Intermittent auscultation is recommended:

- every 15 minutes in established labour
- auscultate immediately after a contraction and for at least 60 seconds
- every 5 minutes in the second stage of labour.

Continuous fetal monitoring should be offered if any abnormalities are detected.

Ensure maternal pulse is palpated and documented to ensure differentiation between maternal and fetal heart rates.

(Reference 5.)

Electronic fetal monitoring (EFM)—definitions

Please refer to local/state policy as some variation in terms (and definitions) occur depending on whether the Royal Australian and New Zealand College of Obstetricians and Gynaecologists (RANZCOG) or the Royal College of Obstetricians and Gynaecologists (RCOG)/National Institute for Health and Care Excellence (NICE) guidelines are used.

For example, RANZCOG defines normal variability as 6 bpm or greater, whereas RCOG/NICE state 5 bpm or greater. The following tables are based on the RANZCOG definitions.

Baseline fetal heart rate (FHR)	Mean level of FHR when stable, excluding accelerations and decelerations; determined over 5 or 10 minutes; expressed in beats per minute (bpm)
Normal baseline FHR	110–160 bpm
Baseline bradycardia	Less than 110 bpm
Baseline tachycardia	Greater than 160 bpm
Baseline variability	The minor fluctuations in baseline; the difference in bpm between the highest and lowest fluctuation over 1 minute

(Electronic fetal monitoring (EFM)—definitions cont.)

Normal baseline variability	≥ 6–25 bpm between contractions
Reduced baseline variability	Between 3–5 bpm
Absent baseline variability	Less than 3 bpm
Increased baseline variability	Greater than 25 bpm
Accelerations	Transient increases in FHR of 15 bpm and lasting 15 seconds or more
Decelerations	Transient episodes of FHR slowing below the baseline level of > 15 bpm and lasting 15 seconds or more
Early decelerations	Uniform, repetitive, periodic FHR slowing; onset early in the contraction and return to baseline at end of the contraction
Late decelerations	Uniform, repetitive, periodic FHR slowing; onset mid to end of contraction, and nadir more than 20 seconds after peak of contraction and ending after the contraction; in the presence of a non-accelerative trace with baseline variability < 5 bpm, definition includes decelerations < 15 bpm

Continued

(Electronic fetal monitoring (EFM)—definitions cont.)

Variable decelerations	Variable, intermittent, periodic FHR slowing with rapid onset and recovery; time relationships with contraction cycle are variable and may occur in isolation Typical features: · presence of two shoulders · sudden fall and rapid return · commonly have V-shape appearance Complicated or atypical features: · increasing baseline rate · decreased baseline variability · slow return to baseline · large amplitude > 60 bpm or down to 60 bpm · long duration > 60 secs (but < 90 sec) · smooth post deceleration overshoots
Prolonged deceleration	An abrupt decrease in FHR to levels below the baseline that lasts at least 90 seconds and up to 5 minutes
Sinusoidal pattern	A regular oscillation of the baseline long-term variability, resembling a sine wave; this smooth, undulating pattern, lasting at least 10 minutes, has a relatively fixed period of 3–5 cycles per minute and an amplitude of 5–15 bpm above and below the baseline; baseline variability is absent

(Reference 12.)

Electronic fetal monitoring classification of features—intrapartum classification of CTG features

Features	Fetal compromise	Action
No abnormal features	Low likelihood of fetal compromise	No action required
Features occurring in isolation: • baseline rate 100–109 • absence of accelerations • early decelerations • variable decelerations with no complicating factors	Unlikely to be associated with fetal compromise	Continued evaluation taking into account the full clinical situation

Continued

(Electronic fetal monitoring classification of features—intrapartum classification of CTG features cont.)

Features	Fetal compromise	Action
• Baseline tachycardia > 160 bpm • Reduced baseline variability (3–5 bpm) • Complicated variable decelerations • Late decelerations • Rising baseline rate • Prolonged decelerations	May be associated with significant fetal compromise	Requires further assessment and action such as addressing any reversible cause; escalation of care; further assessment of fetal wellbeing (e.g. fetal blood sampling)
• Prolonged bradycardia • Absent baseline variability • Sinusoidal pattern • Complicated variable or late decelerations with reduced or absent baseline variability	Likely to be associated with significant fetal compromise	Immediate action required which may include urgent birth

(Reference 12.)

Fetal scalp blood sampling (FBS)

Fetal scalp blood sampling (FBS) is done to measure fetal oxygenation during labour.

Normal values

pH	7.25–7.35
pCO_2	40–50 mmHg
pO_2	20–30 mmHg
Base	< 10
Lactate	< 4.2

Action

Fetal blood sample result (pH)	Fetal blood sample result (lactate)	Subsequent action
≥ 7.25	< 4.2	• Normal FBS result • FBS should be repeated if the fetal heart rate abnormality persists
7.21–7.24	4.2–4.8	• Borderline FBS result • Repeat FBS within 30 minutes or consider expediting birth if rapid change since last sample
≤ 7.20	> 4.8	• Abnormal FBS result • Birth indicated

Contraindications to FBS

- Maternal infection (hepatitis, HIV, herpes simplex).
- Known fetal bleeding disorders.
- Prematurity (< 34 weeks).

(Reference 13.)

Shoulder dystocia

- Manoeuvres in the management of shoulder dystocia are designed to either increase the size of the pelvis or decrease the bisacromial diameter of the fetus.
- Attempt each manoeuvre for at least 30 seconds and ensure that all healthcare providers are aware of the passage of time.
- Continue the manoeuvres until the baby is born or a more experienced operator takes over.
- Careful documentation of all manoeuvres is required.
- Shoulder dystocia is a traumatic experience—ensure debriefing of all involved.

Call for assistance	· Stay calm · Use emergency buzzer/system to call for assistance · Request midwifery, obstetric, neonatal and anaesthetic assistance · Note the time
Change the woman's position (increases pelvic diameters)	· McRobert's manoeuvre (knees to nipples) · Roll the woman over
Evaluate the need for episiotomy	· Allows more room for internal manoeuvres if required

Continued

(Shoulder dystocia cont.)

Apply suprapubic pressure	· May adduct the shoulders and reduce the diameters · Commonly known as Rubin 1 manoeuvre · Need to know position of fetal back to determine the direction of the pressure/rocking
Apply pressure to the anterior shoulder internally	· Insert two fingers into the vagina and exert pressure to adduct or attempt to rotate the anterior shoulder
Attempt to rotate the baby (Wood's screw and reverse Wood's screw manoeuvre)	· Place the fingers of one hand on the posterior aspect of the anterior shoulder and the fingers of the other hand on the anterior aspect of the posterior shoulder · Attempt to rotate the shoulders 180 degrees—rotate the baby anteriorly, then posteriorly to 'screw' the baby out
Attempt to deliver the posterior arm	· Place the hand deep into the vagina · Locate the posterior shoulder · Follow the arm down to the elbow · Flex the arm and sweep it across the chest and face

Shoulder dystocia cont.)

Posterior axilla sling traction	• Use suction or in/out catheter as for sling; some techniques utilise clinician's fingers to provide sling • Fold catheter into loop and thread through baby's posterior axilla • Apply downward traction to sling to deliver posterior shoulder; this creates room for the anterior shoulder to release

(Reference 14.)

Management of the third stage

Women should be supported to choose either active or physiological management of the third stage of labour. When discussing third-stage management plans, consider any risk factors for bleeding after birth.

Active	Physiological
Administration of oxytocic	No oxytocic
Clamp and cut umbilical cord; delayed cord clamping of at least 1 minute (preferably longer) following birth is advised	Cord is clamped and cut after cessation of cord pulsation
Guard the uterus and apply controlled cord traction to deliver placenta and membranes	Placenta is birthed by maternal effort
Palpate uterus to ensure it is well contracted	
Estimate and document maternal blood loss	

(Reference 6.)

Postpartum haemorrhage (PPH)

Definitions

- Primary PPH—occurs within the first 24 hours following birth.
- Secondary PPH—occurs between 24 hours and 12 weeks postpartum.

General considerations

- Prevention is important.
- Early recognition—tachycardia is the most important single warning sign of diminishing blood volume and mild shock; this can often precede a fall in blood pressure, and can be associated with weakness and sweating.

General management

- Call for help.
- Determine cause and treat accordingly (uterine atony—rub up; retained products—remove; genital tract trauma—repair; clotting disorder—restore).
- Resuscitation—**A**irway, **B**reathing, **C**irculation, **D**rugs.
- Intravenous (IV) access—2 large-bore cannulas.
- Blood for cross-match (initiate massive transfusion protocol where indicated).
- Empty bladder.
- Prepare for operating theatre.
  Specific management actions are given on page 59.

Postpartum haemorrhage—specific management

Cause	Management (follow local policy/protocol)
Abnormalities of uterine contraction (atony in 70% of cases)	• Rub up fundus • Consider further uterotonic agents—oxytocin, ergometrine, misoprostol, prostaglandins • Empty bladder • Bimanual compression • Balloon tamponade
Genital tract trauma (20% of cases)	• Inspect for genital tract damage • Repair as soon as possible
Retained products of conception (10% of cases)	• Rub up fundus • Consider further uterotonic agents—oxytocin, ergometrine, prostaglandins • Empty bladder • Manual removal
Abnormalities of coagulation (rare: 1% of cases)	• Identify risk factors • Blood for coagulation studies • Tranexamic acid (as per local protocol/guideline) • Follow massive transfusion protocol where indicated

(References 15 and 16.)

Preoperative checklist

Each facility will have their own preoperative checklist, but there are a number of specific requirements.

General guidelines

- Ensure consent is signed and woman is aware of what procedure is being performed.
- Document last time of food and drink.
- Ensure area of operation has been prepared according to local policy.
- Complete preoperative checklist.
- Gain a copy of most recent test results and put in healthcare record.
- Ensure all healthcare records, reports and documentation are collated.
- Measure vital signs for baseline.
- Ensure sufficient number of identification labels.
- Ensure woman is wearing identification bands.
- Explain to woman what will happen next (i.e. transfer to theatre, what to expect in theatre, where they will recover and when they will return to their originating clinical area).

Caesarean section

- Carry out fetal assessment—auscultation of fetal heart or cardiotocograph (CTG).
- Ensure partner/support person is aware of procedure.
- Assess venous thromboembolism (VTE) risk and apply compression stockings/device (thromboembolitic prevention).
- Check equipment required for newborn resuscitation and immediate care.
- Ensure appropriate personnel are informed if required (i.e. neonatologist).
- Administer preoperative medication as ordered (e.g. sodium citrate).

(Reference 17.)

Postoperative checklist

General guidelines

- Document time of return to clinical area.
- Assess airway.
- Assess level of consciousness.
- Assess operative site and any drains.
- Check intravenous (IV) fluids and IV cannula site.
- Take observations, record and escalate if required (see Vital sign measurement—maternal, p. 15).
- Assess level of pain and address if required.
- Assess comfort and safety (i.e. warmth, no areas of excess pressure on skin).
- Document all assessments and ongoing care provision.

Caesarean section

- Initiate and maintain skin-to-skin contact between mother and baby as soon as possible.
- Assess fundus and vaginal loss frequently.
- Support breastfeeding (or infant feeding) as soon as possible.
- Ensure compression stockings and other anti-thrombolytic preventative measures are maintained.

(Reference 17.)

Postnatal assessment checklist

When assessing a woman in the postnatal period, physical wellbeing, social situation, cultural practices and emotional aspects should all be considered. Often a focused discussion is all that is required. Each assessment or topic discussed involves providing women with information and support.

General wellbeing	· Condition · Fatigue · Vital signs (if indicated)
Emotional wellbeing	· Feelings · Coping · Adaptation · Bonding · Mood
Birth discussion and debrief	· Woman's experience of labour and/or birth · Provide explanation where necessary · Review documentation together · Encourage questioning of experiences · Discuss implications for next birth

Continued

(Postnatal assessment checklist cont.)

Support available/ required	· Partner · Family · Friends · Community · Referrals · Support groups
Nutrition/hydration	· Diet · Fluid intake
Breasts/nipples	· Comfort · Fullness · Damage · Lactation
Infant feeding	· Breast · Artificial
Baby care	· Confidence · Assistance
Rectus separation	· Referral · Postnatal exercises
Uterine involution	· Expected progress · Relate to lochia loss
Lochia loss	· Amount · Colour · Consistency · Odour · Rubra/serosa/alba

Postnatal assessment checklist cont.)

Perineum/Wound assessment	• REEDA wound assessment • **R**edness • **E**dema (Oedema/swelling) • **E**cchymosis (bruising) • **D**ischarge • **A**pproximation • Comfort—ice packs • Healing • Postnatal exercises
Output	• Bladder • Bowel • Continence
Legs	• Oedema • Deep vein thrombosis (DVT) assessment
Mobilisation	• Encourage

(References 5, 17 and 18.)

Recognising and responding to sepsis

Maternal sepsis can occur during pregnancy but is more common in the postnatal period. Signs and symptoms of maternal sepsis can be non-specific and make recognition and prompt management challenging. Some signs and symptoms of maternal sepsis are:

- anxiety and/or restlessness; agitation and/or confusion
- tachycardia—refer to Modified Early Obstetric Warning System (MEOWS) for limits
- tachypnoea —refer to MEOWS for limits
- hypotension—refer to MEOWS for limits
- fever, rigors, hypothermia—refer to MEOWS for limits
- diarrhoea and/or vomiting
- abdominal pain and/or tenderness
- 'flu-like' symptoms
- productive cough
- offensive vaginal discharge
- redness/inflammation of typical postpartum infection sites—breasts, perineum, incision site.

If sepsis is suspected, refer for immediate senior medical support and work as a team to initiate the local sepsis management pathway/protocol. This should include at least the following six key interventions (referred to as the Sepsis 6).

(Recognising and responding to sepsis cont.)

1. Oxygen
- Initiate as ordered/protocol
- Aim to keep saturations within accepted limits

2. Blood cultures
- Facilitate as ordered/protocol
- Collect as soon as possible
- Consider other sepsis investigations—bloods, swabs, MSU, radiology

3. IV antibiotics
- Check blood cultures have been collected prior to administration if possible
- Facilitate as ordered/protocol
- Check for allergies prior to administration

4. IV fluids
- Facilitate as ordered/protocol
- May need a second IV inserted
- Commence fluid balance record

5. Lactate measures
- Facilitate as ordered/protocol
- Serial measures

6. Monitor urine output
- Insert indwelling catheter if necessary
- Commence fluid balance record

(Reference 19.)

As with any emergency management situation:
- work as a team—identify a team leader
- follow local policy and procedures
- report any deviations from accepted limits
- communicate clearly—use ISOBAR tool (p. 93)
- follow documentation guidelines (see p. 92).

Contraception in postpartum women

Type	Use with breastfeeding	Recommended commencement
· Lactational amenorrhoea (LAM)		
LAM	Yes	Criteria for LAM with postnatal women is: • remaining amenorrhoeic postpartum • less than 6 months since giving birth • baby is fully breastfed (no artificial feeds, supplements or solids)
· Hormonal methods		
Combined oestrogen/ progesterone pill ('the pill')/ vaginal ring	Evidence not clear; avoid while establishing lactation	When lactation is established; generally not recommended prior to 6 weeks
Progesterone only ('mini pill')	Yes	Any time after birth
Progesterone injections	Yes	Any time after birth
Progesterone implants	Yes	Any time after birth

· Intrauterine contraceptive devices (IUDs)		
Non-hormonal	Yes	Any time but recommended insertion either in first 48 hours or after 4 weeks
Hormonal	Yes	Any time but recommended insertion either in first 48 hours or after 4 weeks
· Barrier methods		
Male or female condom	Yes	Any time
Diaphragm/cap	Yes	Approximately 6 weeks (once vaginal tone returns); may need re-fitting
· Permanent methods		
Tubal ligation	Yes	Any time; recommendation to wait until some time has elapsed following birth
Vasectomy	Yes	Any time

(Reference 20.)

Supporting breastfeeding

World Health Organization and UNICEF's 10 steps to successful breastfeeding

1	a. Comply fully with the International Code of Marketing of Breast-milk Substitutes and relevant World Health Assembly resolutions. b. Have a written infant feeding policy that is routinely communicated to staff and parents. c. Establish ongoing monitoring and data-management systems.
2	Ensure that staff have sufficient knowledge, competence and skills to support breastfeeding.
3	Discuss the importance and management of breastfeeding with pregnant women and their families.
4	Facilitate immediate and uninterrupted skin-to-skin contact and support mothers to initiate breastfeeding as soon as possible after birth.
5	Support mothers to initiate and maintain breastfeeding and manage common difficulties.
6	Do not provide breastfed newborns any food or fluids other than breast milk, unless medically indicated.
7	Enable mothers and their infants to remain together and to practise rooming-in 24 hours a day.
8	Support mothers to recognise and respond to their infants' cues for feeding.

World Health Organization and UNICEF's 10 steps to successful breastfeeding cont.)

| 9 | Counsel mothers on the use and risks of feeding bottles, teats and pacifiers. |
| 10 | Coordinate discharge so that parents and their infants have timely access to ongoing support and care. |

(Reference 21.)

Immediate care of the newborn

The majority of babies transition smoothly at birth. Immediate care of the newborn at birth should include the following.

Predicting the need for resuscitation/ transition support	Including but not limited to: • fetal—prematurity; multiple birth; large or small for gestation; poly or oligohydramnios; known fetal anomalies/disease; non-reassuring fetal heart rate (FHR) • maternal—diabetes; hypertension; bleeding; infection/pyrexia; substance use; no antenatal care • intrapartum—bleeding; presence of meconium; assisted birth; anaesthesia; narcotic administration; caesarean section not in labour
Equipment prepared (for use if required)	• Safe surface/environment • Appropriate personnel present or immediately available • Resuscitation equipment— ventilation, oxygenation, circulation, fluids, medications • Monitoring equipment—oxygen saturations; heart rate

Continued

(Immediate care of the newborn cont.)

At the time of birth	• Initial assessment of tone, breathing and heart rate—support as required If baby transitioning as expected: • prioritise and maintain skin-to-skin contact (consider partner/support if mother unable) • delay cord clamping/cutting • maintain temperature—dry, skin-to-skin, warm covers • support for initiation of breastfeeding/early feeding • consider environment—quiet, warm, dim lighting, undisturbed skin-to-skin • Observation—Apgar score (see p. 74) • Delay unnecessary interventions—weighing, measuring, routine administration of medications

(References 5 and 22.)

Apgar score

Used to evaluate a newborn baby's condition at birth, usually performed 1 minute and again 5 minutes after birth.

Sign \ Score	0	1	2
Appearance (colour)	Blue, pale	Body pink, limbs blue	All pink
Pulse (heart rate)	Absent	<100	>100
Grimace (response to stimuli)	None	Grimace	Cry
Activity (muscle tone)	Limp	Some flexion of limbs	Active movements, limbs well flexed
Respiratory effort	None	Slow, irregular	Good, strong cry

(Reference 6.)

Newborn screening test

- Blood sample is taken from the newborn baby (usually heel-prick sample) between 48 and 72 hours of age.
- Blood is tested for early detection and treatment of a number of conditions that are rare but important to detect, most commonly:
  - phenylketonuria
  - congenital hypothyroidism
  - cystic fibrosis
  - galactosaemia
  - selected aminoacidopathies
  - selected organic acidaemias, fatty-acid oxidation defects.

Collection procedure

- Gain informed consent from parent/guardian.
- Prepare test equipment/newborn screening test card and record all required information.
- Position baby so foot is lower than body (ideally undertake while baby is breastfeeding or being held).

- Warm the foot—only use approved warming devices.
- Clean and dry the area.
- Puncture the site and wipe away the first drop of blood.
- Gently massage limb above the site (do not squeeze the foot).
- Allow blood to drop into and completely fill the circle—do not touch the card with the foot.
- Allow the card to air dry (at least 4 hours).
- Document collection in appropriate records.
- Follow local processes in regard to sending to laboratory.

(Reference 23.)

Principles of newborn assessment

- Seek consent from parents.
- Ensure baby is in a warm and safe environment.
- Follow standard precautions.

Assessment

Body part	Assessment
Head	Shape, size, marks, presence of caput, moulding, symmetry, bruising
Fontanelles	Should be normotensive
Sutures	Should not be fused, not wide
Face	Symmetry, marks, features
Ears	Patency, skin tags, amount of cartilage, position
Eyes	Shape, opening, positioning, signs of cataracts or sub-conjunctival haemorrhage
Nose	Patent, no flaring of nostrils
Mouth	Palates intact, symmetry
Neck	Check for webbing, swellings, range of movement
Arms	Equal length, tone, movement
Hands	Number of fingers, presence of syndactyly, palmar creases

(Assessment cont.)

Body part	Assessment
Clavicles	Palpate for any injury
Chest	Shape, symmetry, respiratory movements
Nipples	Number, placement
Breast tissue	Presence of
Abdomen	Rounded, soft; umbilical cord clamp secured
Genitalia—male	Descent of testes, swelling of scrotum, positioning of urethral meatus
Genitalia—female	Discharge may be present, observe for urethral and vaginal orifices, observe for skin tags
Legs and hips	Symmetry, tone, movement
Feet	Position, shape, number of toes, presence of syndactyly
Spine	Shape, presence of dimples, hair, swelling
Buttocks	Symmetry of creases, check for dimples or sinuses, observe for presence of anus
Skin	Colour, markings, discolourations

Measurements

Findings are dependent on a range of factors.

Weight	Standard range: 2500–4500 g
Length	Standard range: 48–53 cm
Head circumference	Occipitofrontal—standard range: 31–38 cm

Vital signs

Normal parameters may vary slightly; please check local policies.

Temperature	36.5–37.5°C
Apex beat	110–160 beats per minute (bpm)
Respirations	30–60 breaths per minute

(Reference 16.)

Basic life support

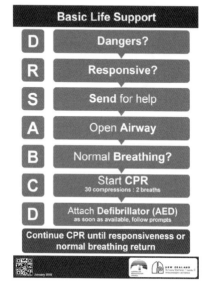

(Reference 24.)

Neonatal resuscitation

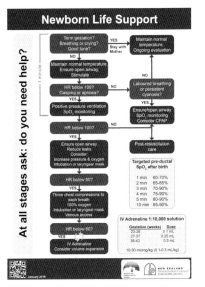

(Reference 22.)

Common abbreviations in medication administration

bd	twice a day
IM	intramuscular
IV	intravenous
mane	in the morning
NEB	nebuliser
NG	nasogastric
nocte	at night
PO	per oral
PR	per rectum
prn	when required
PV	per vagina
qid	four times a day
stat	immediately
subcut	subcutaneous
subling	sublingual
tds	three times a day

(Reference 25.)

Metric system

Length

1 kilometre (km) = 1000 metres (m)
1 metre (m) = 100 centimetres (cm) or
                    1000 millimetres (mm)
1 centimetre (cm) = 10 millimetres (mm)

Weight

1 kilogram (kg) = 1000 grams (g) = 2.2 pounds (or 2 lb 3 oz)
1 gram (g) = 1000 milligrams (mg)
1 milligram (mg) = 1000 micrograms (microg)

Volume

1 litre (L) = 1000 millilitres (mL)

Abbreviations

millimole = mmol

(Reference 25.)

24-hour time

For example:

- 1 a.m. = 0100 hours
- 1 p.m. = 1300 hours.

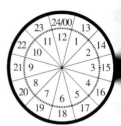

Drug calculations

Calculation of drug doses

$$\text{amount required} = \frac{\text{strength required}}{\text{strength in stock}} \times \frac{\text{volume}}{1}$$

Calculation for infusion rates

The drop rate is provided on all giving sets.
Macrodrop = 20 drops per mL
Microdrop = 60 drops per mL

infusion rate (drops per minute)

$$= \frac{\text{volume required} \times \text{drop rate}}{\text{time in minutes}}$$

$$\text{infusion rate (mL per hour)} = \frac{\text{volume in mL}}{\text{time in hours}}$$

Safe administration of medications

7 rights

- Right person
- Right dose
- Right route
- Right time
- Right drug
- Right documentation
- Right to refuse

(Reference 26.)

Common abbreviations in midwifery practice

AN	antenatal
AFI	amniotic fluid index
APH	antepartum haemorrhage
ARM	artificial rupture of membranes
BMI	body mass index
BP	blood pressure
CTG	cardiotocograph
EBL	estimated blood loss
EDB	estimated date of birth (previously known as EDC or EDD—estimated date of confinement or delivery)
EDB	epidural block
FHS/FHR/FHH	fetal heart sounds/fetal heart rate/fetal heart heard
FSE	fetal scalp electrode
gravid	pregnant
IOL	induction of labour

Continued

(Common abbreviations in midwifery practice cont.)

LMP/LNMP	last menstrual period/last normal menstrual period
LSCS	lower segment caesarean section
multiparous	more than one birth
parity	total number of livebirths and stillbirths of the mother before the current pregnancy or birth
PN	postnatal
PPE	personal protective equipment
PPH	postpartum haemorrhage
primigravida	first pregnancy
primiparous	first birth
PROM/PPROM	prolonged rupture of membranes/preterm prelabour rupture of membranes
SROM	spontaneous rupture of membranes
VE	vaginal examination

Standard precautions

'Standard precautions' and 'transmission-based precautions' define appropriate work practices in regard to prevention and control of infections.

- **Standard precautions**—Work practices that constitute the first-line approach to infection prevention and control in the healthcare environment. Recommended for the treatment and care of all patients.
- **Transmission-based precautions**—Extra work practices in situations where standard precautions alone may be insufficient to prevent infection (e.g. for patients known or suspected to be infected or colonised with infectious agents that may not be contained with standard precautions alone).

Standard precautions involve the use of safe work practices and protective barriers including:
- hand hygiene, before and after every episode of contact with the woman
- use of personal protective equipment (PPE)
- safe use and disposal of sharps
- routine environmental cleaning
- correct reprocessing of reusable medical equipment and instruments
- respiratory hygiene and cough etiquette
- aseptic non-touch technique
- waste management
- appropriate handling of linen.

(Reference 27.)

Documentation guidelines

Midwives are responsible for maintaining comprehensive, accurate and high-quality healthcare records (both paper based and electronic). Ensure you refer to and follow local policies in regard to professional documentation. The following dot points are common to many professional and institutional documentation guidelines.

- Date, time and sign all entries. Signature should include printed name and designation.
- Ensure your documentation is contemporaneous.
- Documentation should be clear, concise and accurate.
- Do not erase entries. Correct all errors with a bracket and strike-through of incorrect entry, and then indicate the error.
- Write legibly in dark ink.
- Chart only for yourself. If electronic records are used, protect your password.
- Use only accepted abbreviations.
- Refer to healthcare service/professional documentation policies.

(Reference 5.)

Professional communication tool—ISOBAR

I = Identification (Hello my name is _____. Am I speaking with _____? I need to discuss the care of _____.)	
S = Situation and status (I am calling to discuss _____ who is currently _____.)	
O = Observation (Her most recent observations are _____.)	
B = Background and history (She presents with a history of _____ and during her pregnancy she experienced _____.)	
A = Assessment and actions (I have attended _____ assessments and am concerned as her _____. I have discussed this with _____ and am requesting that you _____.)	
R = Responsibility and risk management (So my understanding is that you will _____ and I need to _____. Is this correct?)	

(Reference 28.)

Handover checklist

Guidelines

- If you are unsure of remembering all the details, then it is useful to make a note of the salient points.
- Ensure you provide the midwife with key information.
- Do not confuse your handover with irrelevant information.
- Focus on key aspects of care; provide an update and any plan of action.
- Avoid distractions during handover.
- Ensure the person to whom you are handing over is focused on what you are saying.

Details

- Woman's name
- Gestation, number of previous pregnancies/births
- Reason for admission—key presenting problem
- Any significant results of investigations or results pending
- Past medical history
- Significant information about events during current admission
- Key clinical findings
- Social issues
- Tasks which need to be done
- Plan of care

Phone consultation checklist

Document the time and date of the call.
Greet the woman and introduce yourself.
Ask the woman her full name and medical record number.

Document the following

Identification details
Reason for the telephone call
Gestation/estimated date of birth
Fetal movement pattern
Any vaginal loss (i.e. bleeding, fluid)
Any pain
Any uterine contractions
Current social circumstances
- Can the woman get to the hospital if required?
- Does she have someone with her?
- Is she able to organise care for her children if required?
- When is her next scheduled appointment?

Action

Determine the key concern.
Consult with other personnel if required.
Advise accordingly.
Provide follow-up for the woman if required (i.e. ring back in 1 hour), and ensure this is understood by the woman.
Document.

(Reference 28.)

References

1. Australian Health Ministers Advisory Council. *Clinical practice guidelines: pregnancy care.* Canberra: Australian Government Department of Health and Aging; 2019.
2. Australian College of Midwives. *National midwifery guidelines for consultation and referral, Issue 2.* Canberra: Australian College of Midwives; 2014.
3. Clinical Excellence Commission. Standard calling criteria: patient safety programs, http://www.cec.health.nsw.gov.au/patient-safety-programs/adult-patient-safety/between-the-flags/standard-calling-criteria; 2017 [Accessed 12 January 2021].
4. Lowe SA, et al. *The SOMANZ guideline for the management of hypertensive disorders of pregnancy 2014.* Sydney: Society of Obstetric Medicine of Australia and New Zealand; 2014 (updated 2015).
5. Pairman S, et al. *Midwifery: preparation for practice.* 4th ed. Sydney: Elsevier; 2018.
6. Raynor D, Catling C, editors. *Myles survival guide to midwifery.* 3rd ed. Edinburgh: Elsevier; 2017.
7. Queensland Clinical Guidelines. *Obesity in pregnancy.* Brisbane: Queensland Health; 2015.
8. Rankin J, Stables D. *Physiology in childbearing with anatomy and related biosciences.* 4th ed. Edinburgh: Baillïre Tindall Elsevier; 2017.
9. World Health Organization. WHO recommendations: intrapartum care for a positive childbirth experience. 2018.

10. Leap N, Hunter B. *Supporting women for labour and birth: a thoughtful guide*. London: Routledge; 2016.

11. Gray J, Smith R, Homer CSE. *Illustrated dictionary of midwifery*. 3rd ed. Sydney: Elsevier; 2021.

12. Royal Australian and New Zealand College of Obstetricians and Gynaecologists (RANZCOG). *Intrapartum fetal surveillance clinical guideline*. 4th ed. Melbourne: RANZCOG; 2019.

13. Adapted from New South Wales Government Health. *Maternity—fetal heart rate monitoring*. Sydney: New South Wales Government; 2018.

14. The Royal Women's Hospital. *Guideline: Shoulder dystocia*, Melbourne; 2020. https://thewomens.r. worldssl.net/images/uploads/downloadable-records/clinical-guidelines/shoulder-dystocia-guideline_280720.pdf [Accessed 16 January 2021].

15. Royal Australian and New Zealand College of Obstetricians and Gynaecologists (RANZCOG). *Management of postpartum haemorrhage (PPH)*. Melbourne: RANZCOG; July 2017.

16. National Blood Authority. *Patient blood management guidelines: module 5 obstetrics and maternity*. 2015 (Under Review). https://www.blood.gov.au/pbm-module-5 [Accessed 16 January 2021].

17. Johnson R, Taylor W. *Skills for midwifery practice*. 4th ed. Edinburgh: Elsevier; 2016.

18. Davidson N. REEDA: evaluating postpartum healing. *J Nurse Midwifery* 1974;**19**(2):6–8.

19. New South Wales Government Clinical Excellence Commission. Sepsis tools: pathways and guidelines.

https://www.cec.health.nsw.gov.au/keep-patients-safe/Deteriorating-patient-program/Sepsis/sepsis-tools [Accessed 16 January 2021].

20. Faculty of Sexual and Reproductive Healthcare. *UK medical eligibility for contraceptive use (2016).* London: Faculty of Sexual and Reproductive Healthcare; 2016.

21. World Health Organization and UNICEF. Ten steps to successful breastfeeding; n.d. https://www.who.int/activities/promoting-baby-friendly-hospitals/ten-steps-to-successful-breastfeeding [Accessed 16 January 2021].

22. Australian and New Zealand Councils of Resuscitation. *ANZCOR neonatal guidelines.* Sydney: Australian Resuscitation Council; 2016.

23. The Sydney Children's Hospital Network. NSW Newborn Screening Program, https://www.schn.health.nsw.gov.au/health-professionals/statewide-laboratory-services/newborn-screening-program; 2017 [Accessed 16 January 2021].

24. Australian and New Zealand Councils of Resuscitation. *ANZCOR basic life support flow chart.* Sydney: Australian Resuscitation Council; 2016.

25. Australian Commission on Safety and Quality in Health Care. Recommendations for terminology, abbreviations and symbols used in medicines documentation. ACSQHC, Sydney © Commonwealth of Australia, 2016.

26. Gatford JD, Phillips NM, Martyn J, Carey M. *Nursing calculations.* 9th ed. Sydney: Elsevier; 2016.
27. National Health and Medical Research Council (NHMRC). *Australian guidelines for the prevention and control of infection in healthcare (2019).* Canberra: NHMRC; 2019.
28. Australian Commission on Quality and Safety in Health Care. *Communicating for safety*, 2019. https://www.safetyandquality.gov.au/standards/nsqhs-standards/communicating-safety-standard [Accessed 16 January 2021].